# STRENGTH TRAINING OVER 40

## THE 30-DAY NO EQUIPMENT PROGRAM TO BUILD MUSCLE AND FLEXIBILITY

GOLDEN LION PUBLICATION

ISBN: 979-8513795940

# Contents

# INTRODUCTION

# Introduction

Why would you want to be strong at the age of 40? That is an interesting question, and the answer is largely subjective. Only you can answer as to what a stronger physique means for yourself. Strength means different things to different people, especially after you hit the big four zero mark in your life. The reasons to start strength training later in life can vary from the simple desire to have a better-looking body to improving physical flexibility, reducing the risk of disease and injury, and bringing a sense of order and discipline to day-to-day life. All these reasons are important and valid.

Being healthy and happy is at the heart of strength training, giving you peace of mind and better self-esteem along the way. It adds muscle, reduces fat, and elevates your metabolic rate that usually goes down with age. It also reduces stress and anxieties. There is something about physical exercises and exertion that acts as a release outlet to the pressure of daily life. The discipline that comes with maintaining a regular strength training program tends to seep into other areas of life and improve productivity, and the quality of life in general. Moreover, getting into strength training can be an amazing confidence builder, helping you step outside of your comfort zone and seize the day as it is meant to be.

Improving your overall health is a major benefit of strength training, whether you are lifting weights using your body weight for your exercises. Each year the ages of 35, you tend to lose a certain amount of bone mass and can be susceptible to brittle bones that bring many potential risks such as fractures and getting a hunched over posture as you age. Strength training can drastically slow the rate of bone loss that comes with age. When you lose excess weight with aerobic exercises such as walking or cycling, you tend to lose your muscle along with the fat that can lead to a drop in your metabolism as well. Strength training focuses on building muscles, which helps maintain and even boost your metabolism, helping you stay toned and healthy at the same time. The weight loss component that comes with strength training helps keep your LDL cholesterol levels low, hence reducing your risk of cardiovascular diseases which are common among the over forty age group.

There are many pursuits in life that you can do haphazardly and still expect good results. Strength training is not one of them. It requires discipline, and a commitment to see things through to the end. When you work with weights, either you lift that dumbbell, or you do not. There is no halfway. What is important, however, is that you start small and work your way towards your best potential. Strength training is a marathon, not a sprint. Once you are in it, you are in it for the long haul. The good thing is when you experience the exhilaration that comes with proper strength training, you will likely not look back.

Let us guide you through the journey of strength training after 40, step by step. In the pages ahead, you will see detailed instructions for your strength training, starting from stretching, introductory exercises, beginners exercises, and finally advanced exercises with higher training intensities that will help push your limits and help you discover realms in your mind and the body that you had not explored before. You will also see plenty of safety tips and suggestions to make this journey safe and fun for you.

The human body has several major muscle groups that are targeted during strength training. Being familiar with these muscle groups will help you properly follow the exercise mentioned in this book, and later formulate your own training program.

- **Chest** (Pectoral muscles)

- **Back** (Latissimus Dori/trapezius muscles)

- **Shoulders** (Deltoid muscles)

- **Arms** (Biceps/Triceps)

- **Legs and Calves** (Quadriceps, hamstrings, gastrocnemius)

- **Core** (Abdominal muscles)

There are also smaller and muscle groups that further help you break down your strength training process, especially if you are planning to tone your body to become more aesthetically pleasing. These smaller muscle groups include your glutes (muscles in your hips and butt area), delts (muscles that form the rounded corner of your shoulder), and obliques (muscles located on each side of your abdominal muscles). Your workout cycles should be planned in a way that each of these muscle groups is targeted, in order for you to get the best out of your strength training.

Here are few basic strength training terms that you will see continuously in the book and their meanings:

*"Rep"*: A repetition—one completion of a certain exercise. (One

squat, one lunge, one arm curl)

**"Set"**: A number of repetitions before you rest. (8–12 reps of squats = 1 set)

**"Rest interval"**: The time in between sets to rest your body.

**"Intensity"**: The resistance or how hard your body is working during the workout.

**"Program"**: The structure of your strength training. This includes a strategic sequence of exercises that will help you reach your desired goal.

**"Cycle"**: How strength training programs are segmented.

Without further ado, let's start!

"For me life is continuously being hungry. The meaning of life is not simply to exist, to survive, but to move ahead, to go up, to achieve, to conquer."

- Arnold Schwarzenegger

# DIET FOR STRENGTH TRAINING

CHAPTER 1

# Diet For Strength Training

*"Healthy aging is a lifelong guide to your physical and spiritual wellbeing". – Andrew Well*

As we age, the metabolic process in our body naturally slows down. Metabolism is a complex process of biochemical reactions that turn the food we eat into energy, so we can stay active and healthy. Slow metabolic processes mean that our body is unable to efficiently metabolize nutrients from the food we eat. As a result, we tend to lose our muscle mass and it is relatively harder to gain muscle as we get older. Therefore, when you are strength training after 40, it is important to consume food and drinks that help with your metabolism and overall health, while avoiding food that can accelerate the aging process of the body.

## What to Eat and Drink to Help With Strength Training After 40

By the time you are 40, you are hopefully aware of the way your body responds to food. You know your likes and dislikes, your body's natural hunger cues and you have a general idea about how your body metabolizes what you eat. Changing your diet when you start strength training after 40 is less about piling your plate with a bunch of high protein food, and more about adding a variety of food that helps you build lean muscle, with a good understanding of their nutrient profile. Apart from lean proteins, you need a healthy mix of calcium, iron, vitamin c, vitamin B12, vitamin d, and more on your plate to give you the energy to persist with strength training, build muscle, and burn unnecessary fat along the way.

### Lean Meats

Lean meat is a source of animal protein with a lower fat and calorie content. Some meats are leaner than others in general, while almost all the popular meats including pork, beef, and lamb have lean cuts that you can opt for over cuts with higher fat content. When it comes to poultry such as chicken and turkey, the skin accounts for most of the fat content. You can add them to your diet by cooking them without the skin and by trimming off any visible fat before you cook. Rabbit and venison are two other lean types of meat that also have high amounts of iron. If you prefer to stick with familiar meats like chicken or steak, opt for chicken breasts and lean cuts like Sirloin tip side steak or top round steak.

## Fish

Fish is one of the best sources of high-quality proteins and healthy fats, which are exactly the kind of nutrients your body needs when you pass the forty-year mark. Apart from being quite flavorful and delicious without having to add too many ingredients, fish is packed with micronutrients that nourish, soothe and heal your body from within. Some of the important micronutrients in fish that would aid proteins in gaining muscle mass include Vitamin D and B2, calcium, phosphorus, iron, zinc, iodine, magnesium, potassium, and most importantly, omega-3 fatty acids that increase your protein synthesis that fuels your muscle growth. Some of the healthiest fish to eat include Cod, Herring, Mahi-mahi, Mackerel, and Rainbow trout. Wild-caught fish often have more minerals, so a trip to your local fishing spot during the weekends will do some wonders for both your mind and the body.

## Eggs

Being 40 means that you have already settled into a comfortable rhythm of life. Therefore, as you make your transition towards a healthier life and a stronger body, it is always better to amplify the healthy food choices that you had in your everyday meals already—such as eggs. They are inexpensive, widely available, easy to make, and are packed with high-quality proteins and nutrients. Chicken eggs are the closest it gets to a "complete" source of protein. They have all nine essential amino acids that our bodies cannot synthesize from scratch fast enough to supply their demand, therefore we must obtain from our diet. It is, however, important to use a low-calorie cooking method such as boiling or poaching the eggs so you do not add any extra fat calories to the diet.

## Beans and Legumes

With a nice crunchy texture and a pleasant natural flavor to them, beans and other legumes are tiny pods of nutrition that you need to have in your diet. There are a wide variety of legumes you can choose from according to your taste and nutrition preferences, but legumes have been a staple food in many cultures for a reason—they are delicious and are packed with nutrients. Some of the legumes you can add to your diet are beans, peas, lentils, soybeans, and peanuts. They can come in the form of a simple snack to a nice warm bowl of chili that will easily make a meal. Legumes are a great plant-based protein source and have plenty of micronutrients such as iron, folate, magnesium, and potassium. With the high fiber count in legumes, they will help ease the digestion of the high protein meals that you are consuming when you are strength training.

## Tofu

If you are willing to add one new food item to your diet as a part of your strength training, it should be tofu. It is a staple in Thai and Chinese cuisine. This high protein food is derived from soybeans, and popularly has no taste, soaking up the flavors of any topping that you add to it. Some of the nutritional highlights of tofu include containing all nine essential amino acids, just like eggs, making it a great protein option for vegans and vegetarians. Apart from helping out with building muscle and giving you energy for strength training, tofu is also believed to help lower bad cholesterol, and even potentially reduce breast cancer by being a natural binder to estrogen receptor sites in human cells due to the phytoestrogens in tofu that have a similar structure to estrogen.

# What to Eat and Drink to Help With Health After 40

One of the early signs of aging you may experience as you turn 40 is the slower and somewhat weaker response of your immune system. Your risk of getting sick is higher than when you were younger, and it may take a little longer for you to heal from even a common cold. There is also a larger risk to develop autoimmune diseases, conditions in which your immune system mistakenly attacks your body. Oxidative stress or the imbalance between free radicals and antioxidants in your body is another major cause of diseases such as diabetes, cancer, rheumatoid arthritis, cardiovascular diseases, and more. Therefore, it is extremely important to include immune-boosting and antioxidant-rich food in your day-to-day meals.

## Whole Grains

A grain is made of three parts—the bran, the germ, and the endosperm. Whole-grain foods are made of grains that have all three of those parts intact. Refined grains such as white flour have a smoother texture and flavor, but they are devoid of a score of nutrients packed in the bran and the germ. Whole grains have fiber, B vitamins, antioxidants, and a lot of trace minerals such as iron, zinc, and magnesium. While the taste of whole grain food can be coarse to some degree, making the switch from refined grains to whole grains can have a huge impact on your health, especially after the age of 40. Some of the most common whole grains you can easily incorporate into your diet, especially your breakfast and side dishes, include oatmeal, quinoa, brown rice, barley, and buckwheat. Also, make sure you go for whole grain options whenever you buy bread and cereal.

## Nuts and Seeds

If there is one illness that is largely common among forty-year-olds, it is high cholesterol levels, which is a major risk factor for heart disease. The reason for this commonality is mostly unhealthy dietary habits and inactive lifestyles. Cholesterol is a type of lipid which is vital for certain cellular functions in our body. They come in two major forms, LDL and HDL. When it comes to dietary fat, there are also two different forms—"good" or unsaturated fats, and "bad" or trans/saturated fats. Nuts and Seeds, for the most part, contain healthy fats. They are also free of dietary cholesterol, and high in dietary fiber that can reduce the absorption of cholesterol into your bloodstream. As a bonus, nuts and seeds are crunchy and delicious unlike many healthier food choices out there, and you can add them as a topping to many dishes to make them healthier and add an extra level of crunchy texture.

## Leafy Greens

"Let thy greens be thy medicine, and thy medicine be thy greens". Leafy greens are quite literally one of the most nutrient-dense food groups on the planet. They are filled with amino acids, fiber, iron, magnesium, potassium, folic acid, phytonutrients such as beta-carotene and carotenoids, and a whole lot of vitamins. If there is one item of food you are going to add to your diet from this list, let it be leafy green vegetables. Kale is perhaps the most popular leafy green that was recently popularized by celebrities in social media. Kale is rich in antioxidants, minerals, and vitamins, and best consumed raw. If you are not into eating raw greens, Collard greens are a classic option, a thick loose-leaf green vegetable that can be cooked using moist heat until they are tender. There are also microgreens, young leafy greens that are often used as a garnish or for decoration, a great way to improve the leafy green content in your meals. You can grow microgreens in your backyard all year long as well.

## Green Tea

Originated in China, the history of green tea goes back thousands of years. It is one of the healthiest beverages you can consume and slightly nutty bittersweet taste that is pleasant both hot and cold. You can brew a pot of green tea in the morning and taste a warm cup to wake you up, and put the rest in a bottle and drink throughout the day to keep yourself hydrated and help prevent fatigue, stress, and also help improve your metabolism. It is loaded with antioxidants that may improve your brain function and lower your risk of heart disease. Green tea has many powerful bioactive compounds that help treat a variety of diseases. The caffeine in green works as a mild stimulant without adverse effects of coffee such as restlessness and increased heart rate.

## Fresh Fruit

You know the fun old saying, "an apple a day keeps the doctor away". A list of healthy food choices is definitely incomplete without fresh fruit in it. They can instantly elevate your healthy diet and make it more colorful, flavorful, and joyful. Eating whole fruits helps you stay hydrated, control your blood pressure, and even help retain your muscle mass due to the high level of vitamin C they carry. Fresh fruits are also a great source of natural antioxidants, and they have healthy soluble fiber that improves your digestion and lowers the risk of heart disease. An important thing to remember, however, is to limit the consumption of sugary and overly ripened fruits since your body can hold on to the glucose and fructose sugars in the fruit and increase the risk of diabetes. Keep it to one glass of fruit smoothies or one or two cups of fresh fruit per day.

# What Not to Eat or Drink After 40

Avoiding food that can sabotage your fitness journey is just as important as consuming food that can help you. Any kind of workout routine, especially strength training, requires discipline and self-control. Especially if you have been practicing bad eating habits for the better part of your 40 years, it can be difficult to gather the willpower enough to remove your favorite unhealthy food items from your meals. However, prevention is always better than cure, especially at this age. If the kind of food you are eating is making you sick and sabotaging your strength training, it is time to let them go. That said, it is important to know that nobody, not even the dieticians who give you advice, eats perfectly all the time. It is fine to indulge in them as a treat once in a while, ease off the following food and drinks off your day-to-day meals to stay strong and in good health as you age.

## Deep-Fried Food

Deep frying or submerging a food in hot oil is a common cooking method that gives food a crispy texture, pleasant aroma, and flavor. Some of the popular fried foods include french fries, fried chicken, and cheese sticks. However, deep-frying is one of the unhealthiest ways to eat food since they are high in both calories and trans fat. Excess calories can lead to weight gain, while trans fats can significantly increase your LDL levels. Apart from causing obesity and increasing your risk of heart disease, fried food may contain toxic substances such as acrylamide that can lead to life-threatening diseases such as cancer.

If you must deep fry, use healthy oils with high levels of mono-saturated fats and are stable for high-temperature cooking such as olive oil. Using an air fryer is a good way to achieve the same texture and taste of deep frying without the added fat. You can also oven-fry your food, which includes using very high temperatures (450°F or 232°C) in the oven with a small drizzle of oil to get a deep-fried effect with less oil.

## Sweetened Food

Many adults do not think much of limiting their sugar consumption, thinking that if they do not eat sugary snacks and candy that are meant for children, they are good. However, there are many sugar-rich foods and snacks that many adults eat which sneak high amounts of sugar into your bloodstream. Some of these tempting sugar foods include sweetened tea, flavored yogurt, sweet protein bars, cupcakes, cookies, and frozen yogurt.

There are many satisfying alternatives to these unhealthy foods. If you have time, brew your own flavored versions of tea without the added sugar that comes with the store-bought options. You would be surprised to find how easy it is to make blueberry, mandarin, or vanilla flavored tea with zero added sugars. Whenever there is a choice, go for the unsweetened and/or the zero-calorie option of the food. If you like your yogurt with a little added flavor, you can top plain Greek yogurt with fresh or dried fruit.

## Fizzy Drinks

An occasional fizzy drink with popcorn while you watch Superbowl is harmless enough, however, if you are in the habit of drinking soft drinks daily with your meals, turning 40 is a good time to put an end to it. It is the excessive added sugar in soft drinks that can cause harm, especially in the long term. To give some context, an average bottle of fizzy drinks can contain up to 16 teaspoons of sugar. The high fructose syrups in fizzy drinks can only be metabolized by your liver. When you consume them too much, your liver may become overloaded and turn the fructose into fat, which leads to fatty liver disease. Some of the healthier alternatives to fizzy drinks include coconut water, sparkling water, and freshly squeezed lemonade.

## Heavily Processed Food

Simply put, "processed food" includes food that has been pre-cooked, frozen, packaged, frozen, preserved, or changed the nutritional composition in some way. Even the wholewheat bread and chopped apples you buy at the grocery store belong to this category, which means that not all processed foods are bad. Processed foods become bad when they are heavily processed in a way that they have gone through complex chemical processes to change the integrity of the food. Heavily processed food, while easy and convenient to consume if you live a busy life, has many potential adverse health effects. Avoid heavily processed food such as frozen food and pre-made meals as much as possible especially during your strength training

"The clock is ticking. Are you becoming the person you want to be?"

- Greg Plitt, Fitness Model

# STRETCHING
# EXERCISES

## CHAPTER 2

# Stretching Exercises

*"You are only as young as your spine is flexible."* – Joseph
Pilates

Think about that slow stretch of the body you do right after you get up in the morning. How good does that feel? Stretching is a great way to warm up the muscles, get rid of stiffness, improve circulation, and release endorphins that reduce pain and boost pleasure. We do it naturally and even involuntarily since we were babies. In fact, humans are not the only animals who love a good stretch. If you have a cat or a dog, you have probably seen them stretching after a good nap, or even when they are feeling bored after sitting somewhere for too long. Stretching is nature's reset button. It awakens your body and relaxes tight and stiff muscles. Especially as you age, it is important to include stretching in your day-to-day life, since it will reduce pains and help you stay flexible and active.

## What Happens When You Stretch?

Stretching involves deliberately straightening or extending your body parts to their full length, or as much as you are able to extend them. You have over 600 muscles in your body. They are made of fibrous, elastic tissue. Muscle tissue contains muscle fibers, each consisting of a single muscle cell. These fibers can contract, relax, and elongate. When you stretch, your muscle fiber is pulled to its full length. This helps your muscle to realign any disorganized fibers in the direction of any tension or stiffness you have. This realignment is what helps nurse any scarred tissue back to health when you recover from a muscle injury. It also helps heal and recover the muscles that get fatigued often as you age.

When you stretch your muscles, depending on their location in your body, some of their fibers lengthen and some of them remain at rest. The length of your muscle depends upon the number of stretched fibers at any given time. As you learn about the importance of stretching, it is also important to understand the way our brain and the neural components adapt to stretching. When your muscles stretch, the nerve control points that are located among the groups of muscles called muscle spindles also stretch. The function of these muscle spindles is to protect the body from injury and maintain the tone of the muscle. They record the way the length of the muscle changes due to stretching and signals the brain, triggering the stretch reflex which contracts the muscle. When you stretch suddenly, these muscle contractions will be strong and uncomfortable. This is why you have to ease into your stretching.

## Benefits of Stretching After 40

It is natural to lose some of the functionality you enjoyed in your bright-eyed and bushy-tailed younger years once you pass the age of 40. As a part of the aging process, your muscles become less elastic, and you cannot lengthen them as you used to. However, the ability of your muscles to be trained does not stop with age. If you put some time every day into helping them be more flexible, especially with resistance training preceded and followed by a full-body stretching session, you can prolong the time your muscles stay young and healthy. In fact, stretching and strength training are proven to minimize your age-related muscle loss and bone-related disorders.

## Reduces Your Risk of Injury

When your body is warmed up and flexible, it is less likely that you would get injured when you work out or do any type of excessive movement. Stretching helps increase your range of movement, and it also helps decrease any resistance your muscles have, making it easier for you to do more intense strength training exercises. When you stretch both sides of your body, you are also helping remedy any muscular imbalances you have, further reducing muscle cramps and similar painful contractions.

## Makes Your Body More Flexible and Pliable

Aging often makes your joints and muscles stiff which leads to less flexibility. Stretching is an effective way to improve it, since it increases the length your muscle can lengthen, helping you move with ease. When you stretch, your muscles' temporality lengthens, and it comes back to their normal length automatically. When you do not move your muscles much, they become more and more resistant to being stretched. Practicing stretching regularly keeps your muscles ready and improves their elasticity which you can then use for more intense exercises such as strength training.

## Help Reduce Stress

Relieving muscle tension directly impacts your mental state. Stretching, when done properly, is similar to a massage to your sore joints and muscles. A good stretching session often takes time, and it allows you to connect with your body and for your thoughts to slow down. As you relieve the stress that you are carrying on your muscles when you stretch, you are also entering a meditative state that relieves your mental stress as well. Reducing stress from both your body and mind helps you sleep better as well.

## Reduces Age-Related Aches and Pains

Stretching increases the blood flow to your muscles and improves your circulation overall. This helps the muscles to receive more oxygen and get rid of any metabolic waste products that are causing discomfort. It also releases endorphins, a chemical that is produced in your central nervous system that have great pain-relieving effects.

## Improves Your Posture

You are putting your muscles to work when you stretch. You are lengthening them, strengthening them, and basically making them do their job that they do not get to do due to the inactive modern lifestyles that we live. As a result, you will use any tightness or awkward muscle tensions that lead to bad posture. Stretching pulls your spine into positions that help it make better connections with your back, neck, and core muscles, giving you a better posture. With regular stretching, you will notice that you are able to sit up straight with comfort and stand tall with good posture and a straight back.

## Safety Tips

If you are new to working out and conscious stretching that warms you up for the more intense exercises that come after, there are quite a few safety tips that you should know beforehand. If you stretch incorrectly, the chances are that it will do more harm than good.

Here are some tips for safe stretches:

### You Need To Warm Up Before Stretching

Since stretching is considered a warm-up, many people tend to plunge right into stretching before a workout. However, stretching cold muscles can lead to painful strains. Before you start your stretching session, do some light walking, jogging, or using an elliptical bike at low intensity for about ten minutes to warm up your muscles. Just like taffy, warm muscles are easier to stretch!

### Aiming For Pain Is Bad

One of the most harmful beliefs in the fitness community is that if you feel pain, then you are doing a good job. This is not true when it comes to stretching. Your aim should be to feel mild to moderate tension when you stretch. The moment you start feeling pain, hold the stretch. You can try to reset your position carefully and then try again if you wish, but do not try to push through the pain. Do not worry. With constant and consistent practice along with strength training, your flexibility will inevitably improve.

### Symmetry Is Key

Our bodies naturally change as we age, and losing flexibility is often a part of it. When you are getting into strength training after the age of 40, it is always important to keep your expectations attainable. This applies to stretching as well. If you strive to be as flexible as a twenty-year-old ballet dancer when you stretch, it is likely that you will get hurt and discouraged soon. Your focus should be to attain equal flexibility on both sides of your body. When your flexibility is not equal, it can be a risk factor when you are strength training later on.

## Avoid Bouncing

A common mistake that beginners tend to make when stretching is making bounce motions to extend the stretch. This can be harmful and lead to injuries. It's okay to make gentle movements such as yoga which help improve your balance, but avoid rigid and bouncy movements when you stretch. Take your time with the stretch and be smooth when you move while keeping a steady posture. Do not try to rush through your stretching session before the workout. In fact, the longer you take, the less pain and resistance you will feel when you do your strength training.

## Remember To Breathe

Breathe. Inhale and exhale consciously and with purpose when you stretch. Deep breathing lowers stress and stabilizes your blood pressure, which is extremely important before you move onto more intense strength training workouts.

## Upper Body Stretching

Your upper body includes your neck and collar bone area, shoulders and arms, the chest—including breasts in women, back, stomach, hips, and the general waist area. Warming up and stretching your upper body is crucial to avoid any injuries during or after your strength training, especially after 40. The following stretching exercises will help release any stress in your upper body, loosen your joints, and get your blood flowing to your muscles.

## Shoulder Circles

This is an easy upper body stretch to get you warmed up. It helps relax and build muscle tone in your shoulder area, triceps and biceps. You can do it either standing or sitting, and it is discreet enough to do even at your work.

**How to:**

1.  Stand or sit in a neutral position with your back straight. Pull your shoulders back and open up your chest. Inhale deeply and exhale fully. Let your body feel heavy and relaxed.

2.  Raise your shoulders and rotate them slowly forward. Do up to 10 reps, or until you feel a stretch in your triceps. Pause, relax for a moment.

3.  Repeat the exercise in reverse.

## Cross-Body Shoulder Stretch

This is another upper-body stretch that warms up your shoulders, arms, and chest. You can do it while sitting or standing, but make sure you keep your back and chin straight for better posture and results.

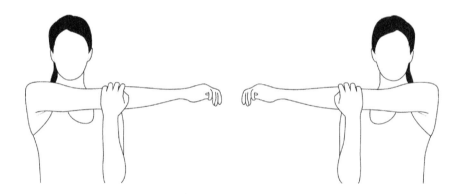

**How to:**

1.  Stand tall or sit with your back straight. Relax your body. Inhale and exhale.

2.  Bring one arm in front of you. Use the opposite hand to grab the elbow, and pull it across your body towards your chest. Move the opposite hand from the elbow towards the shoulder, and gently press until you feel the stretch in your shoulder.

3.  Keep your elbow slightly below your shoulder height and pause for 10 -30 seconds.

4.  Repeat on the other side.

## Lateral Raise and External Rotation

This exercise targets your entire chest area, and better done with a light pair of dumbbells. It is ideal before an upper-body strength training session.

**How to:**

1. Stand tall and let your arms drop either side of you. Take a deep breath and exhale slowly.

2. Grab your light dumbbells and hold them at arm's length.

3. Bend your elbows 90 degrees. Turn your palms towards each other firmly holding dumbbells.

4. Slowly raise your upper arms to the sides until they are at your chest height and parallel to the floor.

5. Rotate your upper arms towards up, and then back, so your forearms are pointed towards the ceiling. Pause.

6. Reverse the movement and return to your starting position. Repeat.

## Lower Body Stretching

Your lower body is made of some of the biggest muscle groups in your body, including your hamstrings, quads, and the glutes on your back. Stretching your lower body helps you do the intense strength training exercises targeting that area, improving the flexibility of what is essentially your body's foundation. If you think of your body as a house, your lower body is the strong foundation that holds the rest of it. By warming up, you can avoid and reduce the pains and discomforts that may occur during strength training.

## Calf Stretch

This is a classic exercise that targets your calf muscles. It does not require any equipment, and even beginners can do it easily and effectively. It is a great way to remove any tension in your lower body before you start your workout.

How to:

1. Stand tall with your feet shoulder-width apart. Relax your body.

2. Step the right foot forward, and keep your left foot firmly on the ground.

3. Bend your right left forward until you feel the stretch on your calf muscles. Do not move your knee past your ankle. Hold for up to 30 minutes, or as long as you can.

4. Switch and repeat.

## Full Body Stretching

A full-body stretch includes stretching and warming up all the main muscle groups in your body including your chest, back, arms, abdominals, legs, and shoulders. Whether you engage in a more intense strength training session later, or simply feel like relieving any stiffness in your body, a full-body stretch is infinitely beneficial. It helps you avoid injuries, and may also help reduce the mobility issues that arise after the age of 40.

## Child's Pose

Inspired by the Yoga pose "Balasana", Child's Pose is a great full-body stretch that uses the muscles of your lower back, inner thighs, and arms. It is an easy and comfortable pose that anyone can do regardless of their age. Apart from all the stretching benefits, Child's pose is great as a stress reliever and an easy remedy for back pain.

**How to:**

1. Kneel on a mat with your thighs perpendicular to the floor, your shins parallel to the floor, and your head facing forward.

2. Slowly put your feet together behind you, with your toes touching each other.

3. Lower your hip backward as far as you can, and sit on your heels. Rest your belly on your thighs.

4. Extend your arms in front of you, and slowly rest your forehead on the floor.

5. Fully give into the long stretch from top to bottom, and let your shoulders and the back fully feel the stretch. Deepen the stretch as much as you can. Relax your body.

6. Hold for up to 30 seconds, or for as long as you feel good.

## Glute Stretch

This stretching exercise targets your glutes and hips. You can do this both before and after your strength training to ease any aches and pains, removing any remaining tension on your back.

### How to:

1. Lie on your back and relax your body. Fill your lungs with a full inhale and exhale fully.

2. Bring your legs up until your toes point to the ceiling, and bend your knees at 90 degrees.

3. Use your hands to place your left ankle over your right knee.

4. Hold your right leg firmly behind your knee, and pull it towards your face. Feel the stretch on your glutes.

5. Hold for 30 seconds. Switch legs and repeat.

## Downward Dog

While it may sound and appear complex, Downward Dog is one of the easiest fully body stretches that you can do, readying your body for strength training. Apart from building strength, this stretch also increases your flexibility and relieves back pain. Make sure you do some initial upper and lower body warm-up exercises before you attempt this full-body stretch.

**How to:**

1. Get into a push-up position, with your legs together and your hands kept firmly on the floor shoulder-width apart.

2. Keep your body straight and your core fully engaged. In that position, slowly move your hips up, forming a V shape with your body, like a mountain. You can slightly bend your knees if you feel too much discomfort.

3. Lower your head and place between your shoulders while keeping your body steady. Feel your body stretch from your neck to your toes. Deepen your stretch by raising your heels.

4. Hold the pose for 20-30 seconds. Return to your starting position.

"Nothing can stop the man with the right mental attitude from achieving his goal; nothing on earth can help the man with the wrong mental attitude."

- Thomas Jefferson

# INTRODUCTORY LEVEL EXERCISES

CHAPTER 3

# Introductory Level Exercises

This chapter is for complete novices to strength training who have never lifted weights before. Also, if you have lifted weights in your early twenties, but have not touched a dumbbell in well over twenty years, make sure you read this chapter to refresh your mind about the basics of weight training. Throughout the book, you will see plenty of exercise options, covering your upper body, lower body, and full body. Using free weights is arguably the more superior method for building strength. However, the book includes workout options both using equipment and without, which you can combine and customize when you put together your own strength training program.

At the end of each chapter, there is a common workout program that calls for training 3 days per week, which is ideal for getting visible results without delay. You do not need to get into that program right away, especially if you are not working out under the supervision of a trainer. Start slowly, and work your way up to that level. The exact days you will be working out is completely up to you, but always leave at least one rest day in between each training day to allow recovery. Your body needs plenty of rest and sufficient nutrition in order to become stronger as a result of your strength training. Be persistent and consistent until these introductory level exercises feel natural and easy by which point you can move to the next stage.

## Basic Training Equipment

Being too overwhelmed by the different types of weight training equipment is one of the biggest reasons people do not get into strength training. However, when you have a clear target and a basic understanding of your capabilities, it is not too difficult to choose your training equipment. In fact, you do not need weights to engage in strength training at all.

Using weights for better resistance is only one type of strength training. You are simply using free weights or other equipment such as resistance bands, tubing, or a weight machine to create stress to the muscles, gradually improving their strength. The same results can be achieved by a no-equipment strength training method such as pilates, which uses your own bodyweight to achieve the same results. If you are new to strength training, however, using free weights or similar equipment can often speed up the results.

Here are some common strength training tools that you can include in your basic kit for introductory exercises.

### Free weights

These are individual objects that are not fastened to anything such as dumbbells, barbells, bars, and weight plates. You can pick them up and freely move around. They come in a wide range of shapes, sizes, and weights. You can start with a small size and weight, and increase as you progress.

## Resistance Bands

These are relatively new in the fitness world. They are bands made of a strong rubber material that can be stretched by putting physical effort. They are affordable, lightweight, and great for strength training beginners and frequent travelers who want a portable tool that will help keep up with their training when they are traveling.

## Weight Training Machines

If you prefer doing your strength training in a gym, you can use a weight training machine such as a Leg Press, a Chest Press, or an indoor rowing machine. They usually have a seat, movable bar, and a cable or a pulley with various weight plates to adjust the resistance and intensity. There are new and sophisticated machines that come with digital features that will give you specific feedback when you are training.

## Exercise Balls

Large inflatable balls that give a bouncy surface on which you can work out, exercise balls give a sense of instability that increases the difficulty level and intensity of your weight training, which leads to deeper use of your back and abdominal muscles.

Here's a basic kit of equipment for you to start with strength training after the age of 40.

- A beginner's set of adjustable free weights
- Mini and full-sized resistance bands

- A yoga mat

- A jump rope

- A treadmill or a stationary bike

**Optional:**

- Adjustable weight bench

- An indoor rowing machine

## Introductory Strength Training Exercises Without Equipment

It is extremely important to note again that you do not necessarily need weights for strength training. The weight of your own body can work perfectly as a resistance method to build strength when you work out. In fact, because they're so simple, exercises without equipment make it easy to prevent injuries. If you're new to strength training and still need some help with the form of your exercises, bodyweight training is much more forgiving than most types of weightlifting. Bodyweight exercises are also incredibly easy to modify to your ability level, which is important especially when you are over 40 years old. They also allow you to develop better balance and control of your body, and better awareness of your physical capabilities in general.

## Upper Body: Push-Ups

Pushups are a stable introductory level exercise that is simple enough to learn quickly, and easy enough to do anywhere. It requires only your bodyweight and targets several large muscle groups and joints. You can start doing your pushups on a yoga mat to be safer at first, but as you make progress in this fitness journey, you will be able to do your pushups wherever you please. Pushups engage your entire upper body, mainly including your shoulders, back, and chest area.

**Muscles most involved:** Pectoralis major, Deltoids, Triceps, Rectus abdominis

### Beginning Position

1. Lower your body on to the yoga mat and assume a high-plant position with your shoulders, hips, knees and feet in a straight line. Keep your hands comfortably shoulder width apart. You should feel the tension of your weight on your palms and toes, but there should be no pain or excessive discomfort. You can start with having your entire body on the ground and slowly raising up to the plank position.

**Downward Movement Phase**

1.  Maintain your steady and straight body position, and lower your chest toward the floor.

2.  Inhale during the lowering movement.

**Upward Movement Phase**

1.  Raise your body up until your arms are extended fully, and come back to the starting position.

2.  Exhale as you come up.

---

<u>Tips and Notes!</u>

Your body should maintain a straight position throughout the exercise to achieve the optimal tension on your targeted muscles. As you inhale and exhale, concentrate and be aware of how your abdominal muscles contract. Once you have your form right, increase your reps.

---

## Lower Body: Lunges

A great introductory level exercise to tone your thighs and hip area, lunges are easy, effective, and can be quite fun if you put on some music to go with it! Even though it is a basic level exercise, you can see lunges being included in a variety of advanced level workout routines due to its weight loss and core muscle training capabilities. Lunges help increase your strength, flexibility, and muscle mass. Moreover, it is great and fun exercise to shape and tone your legs, butt, and the entire lower body area.

**Muscles most involved:** Quadriceps, Hamstrings, Gluteals

## Beginning Position

1. Stand tall with your back straight and your feet hip-width apart. Take a deep breath and relax your body. Make sure your feet are positioned as parallel to each other. Look straight ahead and push your shoulders back.

58

## Downward Movement Phase

1. Step your right foot forward and make it as long as possible while keeping your balance.

2. Bend your knee at a 90 degree angle, as if you are kneeling. Your knee should ideally be directly above your foot.

3. Inhale as you go.

## Upward Movement Phase

1. Return to the starting position by pushing off your right foot and raising your body up. Once you are back in the standing position, your feet should be parallel to each other.

2. Exhale as you go.

3. Alternate your lead foot for each set.

---

### Tips and Notes!

When you do the forward lunge, it is important that your knee does not extend further than your foot in order to keep the stress minimal at the knee joint. If you are finding it difficult to perform the forward lunge due to flexibility and joint issues, you can do the equally effective backward lunge. Maintain the same form at the starting position, and step backward instead of forward. This way, you get to the same lunge position without excessive stress on your knees, which can be a tricky spot after your turn 40.

---

## Full Body: Trunk Curl

Trunk Curl is a highly versatile exercise that targets muscle groups all over your body. It mainly improves core strength but also constitutes flexibility and the mobility of the spine. Since it uses your body weight and flexibility levels, you can be fully in control of how far you'd like to challenge yourself when you do it. Apart from being a great strength training exercise, Trunk Curl helps soothe back pains and tightness by improving your overall mobility. It is, however, important that you take your time with this exercise. Slow, steady, and rhythmic is the way to go.

**Muscles most involved:** Rectus abdominis, Rectus femoris, Hip

### Beginning Position

1.  Lie down on the floor with your face up. Place your hands behind the head, link fingers, and cradle the back of your head comfortably on your hands to maintain a neutral neck position.

**Upward Movement Phase**

1. Raise your upper back off the floor about 30 degrees. This is the "trunk-curled" position that you will maintain throughout the entire exercise.

2. Life both legs off the floor, to a comfortable height. Left your left leg in, and keep the right leg straight.

3. Twist your upper body to the left, maintaining the raised body position and your hands behind your head. Try to touch your right elbow to the left knee.

4. Reverse legs and repeat.

**Downward Movement Phase**

1. Push yourself to complete as many trunk curls as possible with your upper body raised at a 30-degree angle.

2. When it is getting difficult to inhale and exhale, slowly lower your upper body and legs to the floor.

---

### Tips and Notes!

This is a great exercise for your entire body, and especially for your abdominal muscles. Take deep inhales and exhale fully with each twist, and perform the exercise slowly and deliberately for best results. Make sure your upper body and legs stay off the floor during the entire excises. When it's getting too tiring to maintain good form, come back to the floor, take a small rest, and start again. The goal of the exercise is for your elbow to touch the opposite knee, but it can take some time to build up your body to achieve that. Be consistent and push yourself when you feel necessary, but give your body the time to become flexible.

## Introductory Strength Training Exercise With Equipment

Using free weights and other strength training tools when you work out help easily improve your muscle strength, power, and speed. While using your own body weight and lifting weights both help with your muscular endurance and increase your strength, using external resistance often helps with the consistency of the exercise. Moreover, as you move along in your strength training, having external tools makes it easier to level up your resistance than merely utilizing your body weight. That said, both methods are able to target all parts of the body to give a well-rounded strength workout. A well-balanced strength training routine includes exercise both with and without equipment.

## Upper Body: Chest Fly with Dumbbells

If you have not used any tools in your strength workouts before, this exercise is a good option to start. It is a great way to kickstart your muscle growth. You can start with the smallest free weight you have, and work your way towards bigger ones. Due to the lying down position and the free movement of arms, it allows you to work through a wide range of motion. Make sure you do your stretching and have your arms and pectorals warmed up before you start this exercise.

**Muscles most involved:** Pectoralis major, Anterior deltoid

### Beginning Position

1.  Lie down face up on a horizontal gym bench. Relax your body.

2. Straddle the bench securely with your legs and keep the feet flat on the floor. Flex your knees steadily at 90 degrees.

3. Hold the dumbbells on your hands with palms facing each other and raise your hands above your chest, extending as far as you can manage with the weight.

**Downward Movement Phase**

1. Keep your elbows flexed and lower your dumbbells making a wing/flying motion until your arms are extended on either side of you.

2. Inhale deeply as you lower your dumbbells.

**Upward Movement Phase**

1. Bring arms back to the starting position above you, with dumbbells and palms facing each other.

2. Exhale fully as you go.

---

Tips and Notes!

You can slightly flex your elbows as you move your arms for better comfort. As you lower your arms, do not let them fall below your chest or bench level, since doing so would place unnecessary stress on your joints—especially shoulders and pectorals. Make sure your buttocks, shoulders and the head stays in contact with the bench at all times. If you are attempting this exercise for the first time, it helps to have someone spot you to make sure your form is correct.

## Lower Body: Squat with Dumbbells

"Squat" is a staple lower body exercise that helps build strength and power in the hip and butt area and the legs. It is great for the quads and glutes, and incorporating dumbbells into the exercise helps effectively tone the target muscle groups faster. Moreover, doing this exercise with a free weight tool such as dumbbells or kettlebells helps eliminate the right load and tension on the upper back, as opposed to simply using your own bodyweight. Given proper form, squats with dumbbells help target your core, legs, and gluteal muscles, making it one of the best lower body exercises you can include in your strength training routine.

**Muscles most involved:** Quadriceps, Hamstrings, Gluteals

### Beginning Position

1.  Hold your dumbbells with your palms facing toward your body—with your fingers going over the dumbbells, as opposed to underneath it. Your dumbbells should be rotated so your palms face the outside of your thighs.

2.  Keep your feet hip-width apart and stand tall with your back straight.

**Downward Movement Phase**

1.  With your head up and eyes looking ahead, slowly squat down. Your thighs should ideally be parallel to the floor.

2.  Your back should be straight and the weight of the dumbbells should equally go to both your feet.

3.  Inhale as you squat down.

**Upward Movement Phase**

1.  Begin the upward movement by slowly straightening the knees and hips.

2.  Exhale throughout the upward movement.

---

### Tips and Notes!

Maintaining the right form is extremely important when it comes to doing squats. One of the most common mistakes people make when doing squats is dropping their hip area directly downward, lifting their heels, and moving their knees forward too much. These mistakes can cause injuries and even long-term damage if you continue them. Your hip and back should move backward when you come down. You should not move your upper body so the knees go passing your feet, and heels should be firmly on the floor at all times to distribute your weight evenly. When you round your back downwards, do not look down. Keep your eyes forward at all times. This helps maintain good posture and balance.

---

## Full Body: Dumbbell Deadlift

This exercise helps lengthen your muscles and make you stronger and more flexible. It works on all the muscles that you use when walking, jogging, and even simply bending forward as you work or go about your day. Making those muscles strong will make your life much easier and painless as an adult since little aches and pains around your body is often deemed normal as you grow old. With proper strength training, it does not have to be!

Dumbbell Deadlift is a great exercise to improve your grip strength as well, which helps fight effects of aging that are common among 40+-year-olds. It's a great exercise to build muscle and tone your lower back area, legs, hip, and butt. Some of the most irritating aging effects are associated with bad posture. This exercise helps you prevent that from happening, along with reducing tension and pain in your back. Just like many other strength training exercises, Dumbbell Deadlifts help improve your metabolism and lose excess fat.

**Muscles most involved:** Erector spinae, Quadriceps, Hamstrings, Gluteals

## Beginning Position

1. Use the overhand grip to hold your dumbbells firmly on each hand, and stand tall with your back straight.

2. Keep your head up and feet about hip-width apart. You should relax and try to feel comfortable with the dumbbells on your hands. Try to think of them as an extension of your own arms.

3. Flex your knees and hips. Rotate the dumbbells so your palms are facing your legs.

## Upward Movement Phase

1. Rise slowly to a standing position by extending the knees, hips, and trunk.

2. Exhale throughout the upward movement.

## Downward Movement Phase

1. Return slowly to the starting position with the dumbbells on the floor.

2. Inhale throughout the downward movement.

---

### Tips and Notes!

Maintaining straight back posture is the most important thing to remember when doing this exercise. Do not round your back, especially at the beginning of the exercise. The knees should be over the feet rather than extended forward.

---

'The last three or four reps is what makes the muscle grow. This area of pain divides a champion from someone who is not a champion.'

- Arnold Schwarzenegger, seven-time Mr. Olympia

# BEGINNER LEVEL EXERCISES

## CHAPTER 4

# Beginner Level Exercises

The beginner-level exercises introduced in this chapter are a few steps beyond the Introductory Level you just completed. Make sure you are fully familiar and confident with one level before you move forward to the next. At this level, you are familiar with your body and are aware of how flexible you are, how much energy you need, and the intensity at which you can perform your strength training workouts. Beginner level exercises are more complex, and more free-weight movements than the introductory level. Free weights are an integral part of strength training programs, and they help you get into more advanced machine exercises with good form and confidence.

Interestingly enough, using free weights or your own body weight when working out is often more fatiguing than using a weight machine, even when using the same weight. It is due to the lack of pulleys and similar systems that machines used to keep the weight to a fixed amount. When you are using free weights, you need to work harder to maintain your form and technique. On a more positive note, since you are putting more effort with free weights, you do not need to use as many reps as you would need when doing a machine-based exercise.

## Beginner Level Strength Training Exercises Without Equipment

In order to build muscle, you need to challenge the muscle. As you already know, this can be achieved by using your own body weight as leverage. Most of the strength training exercises without equipment that are mentioned here have been inspired by the Pilates exercises. Pilates exercises use your body weight to lengthen, stretch and increase the range of motion of all the major muscle groups in your body. They improve your strength as well as your flexibility and also give you a better command of your body awareness and balance. They make great strength training exercises without the use of any extra tools, they have minimal impact on your joints which make them great for people who are over 40.

The beginner level strength training exercises without equipment that are mentioned in this chapter increase your muscle strength and tone all over your body, particularly of your abdominal muscles, lower back, hips, and buttocks (the 'core muscles' of your body). They help achieve a balanced muscular strength on both sides of your body and enhance muscular control of your back and limbs. They also improve the stabilization of your spine and improve your posture.

## Upper Body: The "Swan"

The "Swan" is a classic strength training exercise that works mainly on your upper body and the back area. It is easy enough for a beginner and has a great impact on someone who is already familiar with strength training. Even if you are using weight training tools in your routine, you can use this exercise as a great upper body warm-up. This is a forward flexion exercise that lengthens your hip flexors and stretches your stomach area. It also targets your arm muscles and improves your posture when you walk and sit.

With consistent practice, this exercise will help you reduce back pain by making your back and upper spine area muscles strong. All of your abdominal muscles stay engaged throughout this exercise, and your glutes and the pelvic floor are also at work. Since this exercise improves your hip joint flexibility, this exercise is great before you do more intense workouts such as Barbell Squat.

**Muscles most involved:** Abdominals, Chest, Shoulders, Glutes, Pelvis

## Beginning Position

1.  Lie down on your stomach on a mat. Take a deep breath in, and when you exhale, connect your pubic bone with the mat below.

## Upward Movement Phase

1.  Raise yourself up by pressing your hands down to the mat, and your elbows pushing back. Your chest and the upper spine should be off the mat and raised in an upward arc—like a swan. Feel your lower abdominal muscles being engaged.

2.  Once you are comfortable with the starting position, straighten your arms raise the rest of your spine and hips away from the mat. Your thighs should be off the mat and be a part of the raised swan pose along with your upper body.

3.  Pause and take a deep breath at the top.

## Downward Movement Phase

1.  Exhale and slowly lower your body back to the starting position. If you have made it to the full swan, start lowering your body from your thighs, then hips, abdominal muscles, and finally your chest.

---

### Tips and Notes!

Make sure you tighten your abdominal muscles and keep them engaged. If they are left hanging towards the floor, you will not get the desired strength training effect. Keep your glutes engaged to avoid any lower back comfort especially when you are starting out. When you twist your pelvis up in the second stage of the Swan, loosen your glutes or they would create unnecessary tension on your back. Your tailbone should be pointing towards the ground at all times for achieving the correct form. When you are in form, your hips should feel fully stretched and when you arch your upper body away from the floor, extend your spine evenly to avoid any discomfort later.

---

## Lower Body: The "Corkscrew"

A good lower body exercise engages all the muscles from your hip to your toes. Even though this pilates-inspired workout does not use any tools, it offers a great challenge especially for your legs and abdominal muscle. Even though it is a beginner to intermediate level exercise, you can intensify it as you get more familiar with the exercise. Both the upward movement phase and the downward movement of this workout work your abs well especially the sides of your body. The rhythmic movement stretches your hip flexors and gives a pleasing massage to your lower body while engaging the muscles. Moreover, as you push yourself to be more intense in this exercise, you can hold your legs together throughout the session to challenge your inner thigh area, which is a hard-to-reach muscle for lower body workouts.

### Beginning Position

1.  Take a deep breath in. Keep your belly scooped in and take your legs up and to the side of your body. Both legs should stay together. Start small and push yourself as you feel comfortable. Your hips should first stay at the mat at first.

**Upward Movement Phase**

1.  With your legs together, draw a circle with your legs with the center being above your belly. Be careful not to lower your legs too much. Keep your upper body calm and stable as much as possible. You can help the movement by lightly pressing the backs of your arms down to the mat to get momentum.

**Downward Movement Phase**

1.  Move your legs downwards on the circle, and take them up completing the circle. Focus on deeply engaging your lower body area. When you are comfortable with making a circle with your hips staying on the mat, you can increase the force and slightly move your hip upwards when you draw the upper arc of the circle to get a nice lower back massage.

2.  Once you complete the circle on one side, you can change the direction and repeat. Continue to move until you have done two to three arcs on each side.

---

<u>Tips and Notes!</u>

Remember that this is a lower body exercise, and consciously engage your entire lower body during the exercise. Your upper body should stay relaxed. As you bring your legs up, the power should come from your core abdominal muscles. Do not depend on the momentum or gravity to swing your legs as you draw the circles. The efficacy of the workout relies on you engaging your muscles to do the work. Do not press your upper body too hard into the mat. Do the exercise for both sides equally, and keep your legs firmly pressed together from your thighs to ankles when you move.

---

## Full Body: The Roll Over

This fun and effective full-body exercise is all about maintaining control of your body and targeting even the smallest muscle groups in both your upper and lower bodies. It effectively trains your back and hamstrings in particular, along with your abdominals. After you do your pre-workout stretching, this workout is a great way to transition to more serious weight training workouts with tools later in your routine. Put on some fun music from the 80s, and roll on!

**Muscles most involved: Abdominals, Chest, Legs, Hamstrings**

### Beginning Position

1.  Take a deep breath in and extend your legs straight up. Your legs should make a 90-degree angle with the floor. They should be kept firmly together, the inner thighs and knees of your legs touching each other. Point your toes toward the ceiling to make it easier to maintain the starting position.

## Upward Movement Phase

1. Tilt your pelvis backward and lift your legs as you slowly exhale.

2. Extend your legs in the side of your head and try to reach them over your head. Press your hands down to help with the pelvis and legs. Pay attention to your core muscles and engage them.

## Downward Movement Phase

1. Lower your legs to the starting position. Take your time and place one vertebra at a time as you lower your pelvis to the mat.

---

### Tips and Notes!

Remember the name of the exercise whenever you attempt it—roll over, not tip over or flop over! The aim of the exercise is not to put your leg over your head, but to strengthen your core. If you try to flop or tip over in the process, you can hurt your neck and back. Relax your neck and shoulders. When you are rolling over with your legs, the weight should be on your upper shoulder area, not your back. At the start, you can use your hands to support your pelvis, but having them on your sides pressed onto the mat is the better form. Always remember, you should use the core muscles when you are raising and lowering your legs, not momentum.

---

## Beginner Level Strength Training Exercise With Equipment

At this stage, you can slowly work your way towards using barbells, the ultimate strength training tool in a gym. A barbell is a metal bar that is able to be loaded with weights. When barbell training, one thing to keep in mind though, is some barbells already come in a pre-made weight and aren't adjustable. Barbells can appear intimidating at first due to their bulky appearance, but once you get familiar with dumbbells, making the transition to barbells is far easier than you would think. It is, however, extremely important that you use the correct form when you do your strength training workouts using barbells. Therefore, make sure you get a professional trainer, or an experienced workout partner to spot you when you are using barbells.

## Lower Body: Leg Extension

You need a lever machine for this exercise. It involves sitting on a padded seat and using your legs to raise a padded bar. Leg extensions are great for your quadriceps—the muscles that are on the front of your thighs. It builds your lower body strength, which effectively decreases lower back issues that can arise as you grow older. Good form is important for this exercise. It is better to have someone to spot you when you do it.

**Muscles most involved:** Quadriceps

### Beginning Position

1. Sit comfortably on the padded seat with your knees in line with the axis. Most resistance machines have a red dot that indicates rotation.

1. Your back should be firmly against the pad of the seat, and your ankles behind the roller pad.

2. Flex your knees 90 degrees and grip the handles for support.

**Upward Movement Phase**

1. Take a breath in, and as you exhale, use your ankles to push the roller pad until your knees are fully extended.

**Downward Movement Phase**

1. Lower the roller pad to the starting position. Inhale as you do so. Take a moment to pause, and repeat the exercise as you exhale.

---

### Tips and Notes!

There are two important things to remember when doing this strength workout. You should always extend the leg until your knees are fully extended. Then, make sure your is straight and against the back of the seat and not arched in any way. Most level machines come with a seat belt to help contract your abdominal muscles so that your back will not arch during the exercise. Remember that you are engaging your thigh muscles, not knees in this workout. You should not feel any tension or pain in your knees. If you are feeling any pain, adjust your range of movement.

---

## Full body: Barbell Squat

As the final full-body workout at this beginner level before moving on to more advanced workouts, this exercise introduces barbells to you. It engages practically every major muscle in your lower body and much of your upper body as well. You are bracing your core, contracting your back muscles and your torse highly engages as you do the squat. It is extremely important that you are maintaining good form in this exercise. Start with a low weight until you perfect your form, and increase the weight only after. You are using more than one joint to perform barbell squats, making it a classic compound exercise. It successfully engages your glutes, hamstrings, quads, and strengthens your joints.

**Muscles most involved:** Quadriceps, Hamstrings, Gluteals

## Beginning Position

1.   Step into the barbell rack and under the bar. Your feet should be shoulder-width apart. Make it slightly wider for

better steadiness if needed. Grip the bar with your fingers going over it.

2. The position of the bar should be on the shoulders and upper back, just below the base of your neck.

3. Stand tall and look ahead. Straighten your knees and lift the bar off the rack.

**Downward Movement Phase**

1. Steady the barbell on your back. Keep looking ahead and your back straight. Balance the weight on both feet, engaging the entire feet throughout the exercise.

2. Squat down slowly, until your thighs become parallel to the floor. Inhale as you go down.

**Upward Movement Phase**

1. Come back to the starting position by slowly straightening your knees and then hips.

2. Exhale as you go upward. After you complete a set, return the barbell back to the rack.

---

## Tips and Notes!

The most important thing to note is not to feel intimidated by the barbell. Start with the lowest weight until you feel comfortable and you are confident with your form. Have a competent trainer spot you until they are satisfied with your form. Make sure the bar is not too high on your neck. Do not try to do too much too fast. Take your time.

---

'What hurts today makes you stronger tomorrow.'

- Jay Cutler, pro bodybuilder and four-time Mr. Olympia

# ADVANCED LEVEL EXERCISES

## CHAPTER 5

# Advanced Level Exercises

After completing your introductory and beginner level exercises, now you have gotten into a steady strength training routine. You are more knowledgeable about using resistance exercises to improve your endurance, and you have a stronger and more flexible body. At this point, you are prepared to start a true strength program with advanced workouts. If there is one thing to keep reminding yourself of at this level, it is that technique is key. You need proper form and technique to avoid any injuries from happening, and without it, your entire process would be stagnated and unsuccessful.

Practise makes perfect, and more importantly, practice makes your results permanent. You are likely experiencing improvements not only in your physical appearance and energy levels but also in your mind. You are more focused, attentive, confident, and motivated. Your introductory and beginner levels are better done with a qualified trainer to spot you, guide you, and perfect your technique. If you continue with poor technique, it will ultimately cause irreversible damage, and make it difficult to correct your mistakes. Always listen to your body. Learn how to understand the difference between the pain that is asking you to stop what you are doing, and the strain that is showing you that you are making progress. Take your time. You are running a marathon, not a sprint!

## Upper Body: The "Rising Swan"

This is an advanced version of the "Swan" you did at the Beginner level. The Rising Swan further engages your upper body. It opens up your front chest area, expands and stretches it, and works your abdominal muscles, quadriceps, and hips. When a person gets older, they naturally tend to sit down more than they used to. The Rising Swan is a good exercise to improve the posture when sitting and to heal any tightness or pain caused by prolonged sitting. It also strengthens your abdominals, pelvic floor, and glutes. If you are a jogger or a runner, this exercise improves your hip joint flexibility. It will also make it easier for you to do workouts with equipment by improving your flexibility.

### Beginning Position

1. Lie down comfortably on your stomach. Lift your upper body until your belly button is lifted away from the mat. This position should be maintained throughout the website, with your abdominal muscles lifted away.

**Upward Movement Phase**

1.  Take a deep breath in. Press your forearms down on the mat and lengthen your spine resembling the upper body of a swan. Create a long upward arc from your body. Your head should be in line with your spine, and the elbows should be firm and closer to the body. Push your tailbone toward the map and make sure the hip stays on the map.

**Downward Movement Phase**

1.  Release your upper body arc as you exhale, but keep your abdominal muscles lifted. Return your torso to the mat slowly and sequentially.

2.  Maintain a deep, even, and flowing breath that supports the movement throughout.

3.  Once you complete a set, finish by bending your knees and the rounded and rested on your thighs.

---

<u>Tips and Notes!</u>

How far you stretch your body and how high you raise the torso is completely up to you. Be mindful of all the muscle groups that are engaging. It is a must to properly do your warm-up stretches before you do this exercise. Lifting of the torso should not be done by putting weight on your arms. Let your core muscles do that. Once you are fully familiar with the workout, you can even lift your hands off the mat briefly for a more intense effect.

---

## Lower Body: The "Mountain Climber"

Think of the difficult but extremely rewarding task of climbing a mountain, and imagine that the mountain is the floor. That's the concept behind this workout. It is performed in a plank position, a challenging strength workout that is simple yet highly effective. You are bringing your knees to the chest and back as if you are walking or running against the floor depending on the speed at which you do it. Just like other workouts that use body weight as resistance, you have to be highly conscious about which muscle groups that you target when doing this exercise. Once you feel confident about the basic workout, you can add variations and engage the entire body as well.

### Beginning Position

1. Get into a plank position, making sure to distribute your weight evenly between your hands and your toes.

2. Check your form—your hands should be about shoulder-width apart, back flat, abs engaged, and head in alignment.

**Upward Movement Phase**

1. Pull your right knee into your chest as far as you can.

2. Switch legs, pulling one knee out and bringing the other knee in.

**Downward Movement Phase**

1. Keep your hips down, run your knees in and out as far and as fast as you can. Alternate inhaling and exhaling with each leg change.

<u>Tips and Notes!</u>

Proper form in this exercise is a must not only to maximize its effectiveness but also to prevent any injury. A common mistake that can happen is bouncing on toes when performing the climbing move. While it may feel like you are working harder as you bounce, it leads to not getting proper core engagement for the move. Also, when you bring the knees towards the chest, you have to complete the movement by letting the toes touch the ground.

## Full Body: The "Boomerang"

This is an advanced strength training exercise that combines several Pilates moves that are used in classic mat sequences. It uses several skills that creates a flawless sequence of moves that targets muscle groups all over the body. It is easier to remember this workout like choreography and you can put on your favorite music to make the experience even more fun and enjoyable. The "Roll Over" exercise you did in the earlier level is also a part of this exercise. Once you complete this full workout from the beginning to the end, it's quite possible that you would work up a good sweat in the end. When done properly and practised consistently, this exercise will build flexibility and strength throughout your core area and the back, giving you good posture. It is also great for toning and strengthening your legs and improving your overall balance and coordination of the body.

### Beginning Position

1.  Sit tall on your sit bones with your legs outstretched and crossed.

2.  Seal your legs together and feel the sense of midline moving from your legs up your spine and through the top of your head. Maintaining that feeling as you move will help you keep the boomerang shape and give you a line of energy to move along.

3.  Place your hands on the mat by your sides.

4.  Take your body into a Pilates C-curve.

## Upward Movement Phase

1.  Exhale: Deepen your C-curve and roll back, taking your crossed legs overhead as you would in the rollover exercise. Your body has taken a boomerang shape and will keep that shape through the exercise.

2.  You are between your shoulders; the backs of your arms press against the mat, adding stability.

3.  At the top of the roll, uncross your legs and re-cross with the other leg on top.

## Downward Movement Phase

1.  Inhale: Bring your whole body up to the teaser position. Keep your boomerang shape. This is an abdominal control move—not a drop of the legs and then a regroup.

2.  Continue the inhale as you hold your teaser shape and sweep your arms around to the back. Keep your arms high and perform it with your palms up.

3.  Exhale: Stay in control of the shape as you smoothly let your legs come down and sweep your arms wide to the sides.

4.  Continue your exhale as you let your arms come all the way to the front (shoulders down, neck long) as you curve over your legs and prepare to begin the sequence again.

5.  Start from here with a deep scoop of the belly. Your hands can come back to the mat along your sides to help you.

## Upper body: Barbell Bench Press

A classic high power upper body strength training exercise, the bench press highly effective and versatile in its benefits. It increases your upper body push strength, which is an important factor and skill for all strength training exercises. It tones and builds up your pecs, which will make your body look youthful and attractive. It also gives a nice shredded appearance to your anterior muscles that are wrapped around your rib cage, makes your delts stronger and toned, and strengthens and builds up your triceps. All in all, the barbell bench press is as close as it gets to a perfect upper body strength training exercise.

**Muscles most involved:** Pectoralis major, Anterior deltoid, Triceps

### Beginning Position

1. Lie supine with the legs straddling the bench, the knees flexed at 90 degrees, and the feet flat on the floor.

2. Grasp the barbell in an overhand grip with the palms facing away and press the bar until the arms are fully extended above the chest.

**Downward Movement Phase**

1. Lower the bar slowly and evenly to the chest.

2. Inhale throughout the lowering movement.

**Upward Movement Phase**

1. Press the bar upward evenly until the arms are fully extended.

2. Exhale throughout the pressing movement.

---

<u>Tips and Notes!</u>

Before you attempt this exercise, make sure your bench has secure uprights to hold the bar. You also need a trained spotter to get you through the exercise safely and effectively. Your head, shoulders, and upper back should be in contact with the bench at all times while performing the exercise. Both your feet should be firmly on the floor. Engage your chest and upper body muscles to move the bar, without depending on the momentum.

---

## Lower body: Barbell Heel Raise

This exercise is a variation of the standard squat. Raising the heels during the movement increases the depth of the squat while building lower-body strength. This is also a good alternative exercise for those who cannot perform the standard squat due to low hip flexibility.

**Muscles most involved:** gastrocnemius, soleus

### Beginning Position

1.  Remove the barbell from the rack and assume a position with the bar on the shoulders; then move the bar to the base of the neck.

2.  Place the balls of the feet on a stable elevated surface approximately 2 inches high, about hip-width apart and parallel to each other.

## Upward Movement Phase

1. Keep the head up, eyes fixed straight ahead, shoulders back, back straight, and weight on the balls of the feet throughout the upward and downward movement phases of this exercise.

2. Rise up slowly onto the toes while keeping the torso erect and the knees straight.

3. Exhale throughout the upward movement.

## Downward Movement Phase

1. Lower the heels as far as is comfortable while keeping the torso erect and the knees straight.

2. Inhale throughout the lowering movement.

---

### Tips and Notes!

Because of the relatively short movement range, you should hold the fully contracted position momentarily on each repetition.

---

## Lower body: Barbell Front Squat

The squat exercise, in general, provides numerous health benefits. Squats build strength and can improve athletic performance in healthy, young adults.1 But they have also been shown to provide benefits to older adults who are trying to preserve physical function and lung capacity. Many advanced exercisers use squat variations to achieve substantial gains at the gym. There are differing opinions about whether the front squat or the back squat is a better way to work the lower body. There has been some (but not a lot) of research comparing the two exercises. Each has its own place in a comprehensive weight training program. But the front squat has a few unique advantages.

### Beginning Position

1.  Begin to lower the body into a deep squat with the weight descending down. Keep the spine long and the back tall and upright. You'll notice that the back stays almost completely vertical as you descend, unlike a traditional squat where the torso leans slightly forward.

2. Your hips stay under the bar (rather than floating behind the bar in a traditional squat) even as your glutes continue to lower down below knee level. You'll also notice that the knees extend further out in front and the ankles flex more than in a traditional squat.

**Downward Movement Phase**

1. Keep the heels on the ground and your weight centered over the middle of your feet as you continue to descend. Try not to shift forward into the balls of the feet or back into the heels.

2. At the lowest position, your hamstrings will nearly touch the back of the calves. Keep elbows lifted at bar height (if possible) and chest upright to prevent the bar from rolling forward.

**Upward Movement Phase**

1. Reverse the squat in a slow, controlled manner with the hips and knees extending simultaneously. Continue lifting until the body is back at the starting position.

---

### Tips and Notes!

If your wrists are not flexible, you will have a hard time keeping the elbows lifted. But if the elbows drop down during the squat, you run the risk of the bar rolling forward and off of the chest which can be a safety hazard. As mentioned, grip and elbow placement are key for proper form and safety. If you work out in a gym, it's easy to assume that the grip used by your fellow gym-mates is the right grip for you. But for this exercise, personalization is important. Use the grip that works best for your body so that you can keep your elbows elevated and chest lifted. Ultimately, it's far more important to keep the barbell in place as you squat than it is to look like everyone else in the gym.

---

"No citizen has a right
to be an amateur in
the matter of physical
training... what a disgrace
it is for a man to grow
old without ever seeing
the beauty and strength
of which his body is
capable."

- Socrates

# CONCLUSION

# CONCLUSION

A muscle is like a car—if you want it to run well, you have to warm it up! There are numerous health benefits associated with proper muscle building and strength training, especially for older adults. Due to the intimidating and confusing nature associated with strength training and the many different weights and tools used in exercises, many people over the age of 40 are reluctant to start strength training on their own. Acquiring a better understanding of getting into a sensible strength training program is important to developing a good strength training program.

Many people assume that working out is mainly about getting a more aesthetically pleasing physique. Therefore, while many in their twenties and thirties do have at least a basic working out routine in their everyday life, it tends to fade away as a person gets older. In reality, however, the need for consistent exercises increases with age, since metabolism has a direct correlation with physical activity, and it goes down during the aging process. Having too little muscle and too much fat on the body as an adult can lead to a plethora of health challenges after 40 such as cardiovascular disease, diabetes, osteoporosis, and even cancer. Strength training, in particular, has a great many advantages to an aging body. Aside from increasing metabolic rate, strength training helps replace muscles, reduce fat, decrease lower-back discomfort and arthritic pain varieties that are common among people after the age of 40, as well as boosting self-confidence.

Nutrition plays a great part in starting and maintaining a healthy strength training routine. Just like any other strength trainer or someone who engages in a muscle-building activity, adults over 40 also benefit from plenty of good proteins in their diet. A sound diet should go hand in hand with strength training exercises for them to work since a consistent workout program requires a large amount of both physical and mental energy. A good diet for strength training consists of generous amounts of lean meats, whole grains, fish, eggs, leafy greens, and more nutritious food. It is also equally important to avoid sugary snacks, deep-fried food, fizzy drinks, and other similar unhealthy food, which is anyway a necessary change in one's diet particularly after 40.

Getting into strength training is a gradual process. It should be treated more like a marathon, not a sprint. The introductory, beginner, and advanced level exercises mentioned in this book are to be considered as a guide that points you in the right direction, rather than a set program that is meant to be followed by everyone. Regardless of which stage you are in, there is no "perfect program" or a template that you can follow in order to get optimal results. It is all about trying out safe and proven exercises and finding out what works the best for you.

The type of exercise you do often does not matter as much as the level of effort and consistency that goes into it. The workouts mentioned in this book are solid and reliable and would give you a great start on your fitness journey. If you commit to them and persist with your training, you will eventually figure out the best program that works specifically for you. Good luck!

# REFERENCES

# REFERENCES

- https://www.ncbi.nlm.nih.gov/pmc/articles/PMC4193807/
- https://www.prevention.com/health/a20487687/10-ways-your-diet-should-change-after-40-according-to-nutritionists/
- https://web.mit.edu/tkd/stretch/stretching_2.html
- https://legionathletics.com/muscle-groups

# SHARE YOUR EXPERIENCE WITH US ON AMAZON BY LEAVING A QUICK 30-SECOND REVIEW

# DISCOVER MORE FROM GOLDEN LION PUBLICATIONS ONLY ON AMAZON

Printed in Great Britain
by Amazon

65152976R00071